How Get Rid Of Headache Naturally

The Migraine And Headache Program

John Zager

Table Of Contents

Disclaimer Notice

All the material contained in this book is provided for educational and informational purposes only.

No responsibility can be taken for any results or outcomes resulting from the use of this material. While every attempt has been made to provide information that is both accurate and effective, the author does not assume any responsibility for the accuracy or use/misuse of this information.

In practical advice books, like anything else in life, there are no guarantees of specific results. Readers are cautioned to rely on their own judgment about their individual circumstances to act accordingly.

This book is not intended for use as a source of professional health advice. All readers are advised to seek services of competent professionals the medical field. Readers acknowledge that the publisher is not engaging in rendering legal, financial or professional advice.

Introduction

There are many different types of headaches. Some of which include tension headaches, cluster headaches, migraines, allergy and sinus headaches, and common headaches. All are uncomfortable, maybe throbbing, and can easily being distracting because of the pain from the headache.

Everyone in their life will experience some type of headache. Having them occasionally isn't a big deal. However, having a headache is not something that is fun to have when you have to get through the day. Having a headache can significantly slow you down and prevent you from doing the things you need to do. Therefore, we will be covering some different natural ways to avoid headaches and things you can do once you have them.

Headaches are a good indicator that your body is missing something. They can be caused by a variety of things like stress, anxiety, allergies, fatigue, low blood sugar, hormone imbalance, drugs you are taking, eye-strain, dehydration, and more.

What "Natural" Means

There are many different types of natural treatment options. The term "natural" simply means "without chemical medicine," and this opens up hundreds of different doors that you can choose from to help you reduce the intensity and frequency of your headaches naturally.

Types of Headaches

Common headaches occur when you're having pain in your head and there isn't due to an illness or allergies. Episodic headaches happen just every occasionally. They general last a short time like ½ hour up to several hours. When they become chronic is when they are more consistent. They occur most days during a month period and they can last for days at a time.

Tension headaches: You may have pain in your head, but you will also have tenderness in and around your neck, scalp, and forehead. Shoulder muscle pain may also occur. Tension headaches are generally triggered by stress. It is good if you can figure out what the triggers are for your headaches. This will make finding a successful natural treatment so much easier.

Cluster headaches are generally a piercing pain. They will occur around or behind one eye or on the side of the face. They are generally occurring in a series. They may last 15 minutes to a few hours. People who suffer from these headaches can experience one to four of these a day.

Generally though, they occur around the same time each day. Once one headache resolves itself in the cluster the next is shortly to follow.

Migraines are an intense, pulsating pain deep within your head. These headaches can last for days. Migraines can limit your ability to carry out your daily normal routines. They throb and are usually one sided. People with migraine headaches are often light and sound sensitive. It is not unusual for nausea and vomiting to occur.

Some migraines will have visual disturbances. This may happen before the migraine even starts. It could be flashing lights, zig zag lines, stars, or blind spots. Auras can also occur. Some symptoms of these headaches include tingling on one side of your face or in one arm and some may experience trouble speaking.

Environmental factors can trigger migraines also. Things like sleep disruption, hormone fluctuations, and chemical exposure are common migraine triggers for some people. They can also be caused by stress, anxiety, sleep deprivation and hormonal changes.

Allergy and sinus headaches are generally focused in your sinus area and in the front of your head. People can have pain, tightness, and pressure in the forehead, behind the eyes, and on either or both sides of the nose.

Sometimes the simple movement of bending over can make these headaches worse. People who have chronic seasonal allergies are susceptible to these types of headaches.

Sinus headaches can also be a sign of a sinus infection, so sometimes a trip to the doctor may be needed. To help with sinus headaches you must thin out the mucus that builds up and causes the sinus pressure.

Stress is a huge cause of headaches. Having ways to relieve your stress throughout the day is something that will make you feel good as well.

Environmental Causes

Environmental issues can cause headaches. Limiting exposures to known environmental allergens may help reduce your sinus headache. Heavy perfumes or other smells are a trigger for many people.

Being aware of what you are around, asking family members not to wear such heavy items, etc. may help reduce headaches brought on by these items. Barometric pressure changes that happen quickly can also cause headaches. Do your best to be aware of these possible upcoming changes.

Although you cannot avoid them altogether, having a plan in place on days this may happen may help you prevent or quickly treat your headache.

Allergies are easy to learn about and start treating. If you are unaware of what you are allergic it may be helpful to start going to an allergy doctor. Once you know what you are allergic to you can start to eliminate those things in your life to the best of your ability. Starting to rid yourself of known triggers will help begin to relieve symptoms.

Natural Remedies for Headaches

<u>Diet</u>

Your diet can be a cause of headaches. You may not even know what you might be eating that is triggering it! Start by keeping a food journal. Think about what you eat.
You need to make sure that you watch what you eat. This may be the best thing you can do to prevent your headaches. This will help you spot trends and may help you figure out what you need to eliminate in your diet if you suspect it to be a trigger food.

Skipping meals and eating at different times can bring on migraines, so make sure you eat the needed meals each day and eat around the same time you normally would. Consider doing a gluten free diet. Try eliminating it for three weeks and see how you feel.
After the elimination you can start to add one food back each time, keeping track of how you feel. Some people just have a gluten sensitivity and may find that just cutting back on the amount of gluten they ingest daily will help to lower the amount of headaches they get.

Herbs for Headaches

Herbs can be helpful for reducing and possibly even eliminating headaches. Fever few is one that helps to reduce the frequency of migraines, as well as the awful symptoms that can go along with them, such as nausea, vomiting, and light sensitivity.

Butterbur is an herb that is known to reduce inflammation. It is also known for its possibility of being a beta blocker, which results in normal blood flow to the brain. Basil is known for its ability to treat headaches naturally. It also has many analgesic benefits. It is a great muscle relaxant which can help with the tight muscles and tension headaches.

Try taking 4 fresh basil leaves in a large cup of boiling water. Let steep, you can add a taste of honey to it also. Drink slowly. If drinking basil tea isn't your thing you can also inhale the steam from the cup after boiling basil in a pot of water.

Light and Headaches

Lighting can trigger headaches and migraines. Bright or flickering lights (such as computer and television screens) or florescent lights can be a trigger for many people.

Wearing sunglasses and a hat or visor to shade your eyes may help. In addition, turning down the lighting on your electronic devices may help.

Supplements

Magnesium is something that our body uses a lot of, especially in high stress situations. Many foods that we buy are stripped of this nutrient, so it may be necessary for you to take a high-quality supplement of magnesium or buy it in oil or spray form.

Magnesium may help reduce the frequency of headaches. Dietary sources of magnesium include whole grains, broccoli, squash, leafy greens, dairy products, beans.

Exercise

Exercise can sometimes trigger headaches. Make note when this happens. If you have talked to your doctor about it and have been cleared to exercise, then still do so. Mild exercise is good for your entire body. Even a 15-minute daily walk is better than nothing. Having the right exercise in your life is going to make you feel your best and get your blood pumping the way it should be. Exercising can also help to reduce stress, a major cause of headaches. Yoga is a wonderful way to incorporate physical activity and stretching into your daily life. Yoga is great for controlling your breathing and creating relaxation. Yoga is also a great prevention for headaches.

Self-Care

Sleep can be a big contributing factor to any headaches. Too much sleep, too little sleep, poor sleep, and irregular sleep can all trigger migraines. If you are having a difficult time getting to sleep, try looking at your life patterns. Sleep can be a great preventative of headaches when you get good quality and the amount you need. Limit caffeine and exercise for a little bit before bed.

Eliminate watching TV and reading on a computer or handheld device at least an hour before bed. Do not use electronics to relax. Eliminate extra noise, sound, and lights from your sleeping area.

Make sure your sleeping area is peaceful. Make a nighttime routine. Try to go to bed around the same time every night and get up around the same time every morning.

Schedule and routines can help keep headaches away. Our bodies thrive on normal. Make a normal for yourself. Aim to get up at the same time every day. Aim to go to bed around the same time every night. Incorporating an evening routine will be helpful.

Your body will begin to get used to it and understand what it is supposed to do next. Have an eating schedule. When your body gets used to having its blood sugar at a certain level and you decide not to eat for two extra hours the blood sugar will go down and this can cause headaches and many other unpleasant symptoms.

Water consumption is so important for the human body. All our organs thrive off of having enough water in the body. Frequent dehydration can cause a severe headache and migraine.

Try to avoid things like alcohol and caffeine, as these are all very dehydrating and can leave you with a painful headache. Set reminders for yourself daily if needed to drink more water. Some fruits and vegetables also help to hydrate you because some are known to contain 90% or more of water.

Try adding some of these to your diet daily: cucumbers, zucchini, eggplant, spinach, watermelon, cantaloupe, oranges, grapefruit, and cabbage.

Taking care of your body, eating right, getting plenty of rest and exercising are all things that are going to help you prevent headaches in your everyday life.

Resting or sitting in a darkened room can help relieve symptoms of headaches and migraines. Closing your eyes and letting your neck, back and shoulders relax will also help to reduce symptoms of headaches.

When you have headaches, it is much harder to perform at your job and life well. It makes it harder on relationships with family and friends.

There are simple things you can do to help prevent headaches and treat headaches naturally. Taking a detox bath every once in a while, may be of great relief to you. A detox bath is great for cleansing your body and ridding it of toxins that can make you sick. A detox bath recipe is included in this report. Massage can be used to help treat headaches that arise. You can have someone give you a massage or you can massage certain parts of your body yourself.

Try rubbing peppermint and lavender essential oils mixed with your favorite carrier oil into your temples and the back of your neck to relieve a headache. Eucalyptus essential oil and peppermint essential oil combined with your favorite carrier oil may be good for tension headaches. You can rub this combination onto your temples, forehead and wrists. It will help alleviate stress and reduce tension. Try simple things like massaging each fingertip and massaging your skull.

Pressure points can be a great way to treat many aliments naturally. Pressure points can be found throughout your entire body. A pressure point is a sensitive spot on your body that is stimulated when pressure is applied.

You can find pressure points for headaches in your hand between your thumb and index figure. You can apply gentle pressure to this area daily. Below the base of your skull. There are two points at the base of your neck, behind your ears.

You can apply pressure to these points with your thumbs. In between your eyebrows above your nose, and many more spots. Apply pressure between the eyebrows with your thumb. Using pressure points can he highly effective for some people. Stretching is another great way to help reduce painful headaches. When we stay in one position for a long period of time we tend to get stiff and this leads to tension in our bodies which helps create headache symptoms.
Try to remember when sitting in a position for a long time at your desk, or on your phone to take a break every thirty to sixty minutes. Stretch and move. Your circulatory system will thank you.

Some simple stretches that you can do for your neck and body with help reduce the intensity of a headache. Try doing this simple neck movements: Move your chin up and down (like you are saying yes), then start moving it left and right (like you are saying no), start bending your neck sideways going slowing to each shoulder.

Lastly, you can rotate your neck slowly in a clockwise and then counter clockwise position. This will help your neck muscles start to relax and reduce tension in your neck.

Recipes

Detox Bath

1 Cup baking soda

Baking soda is great for killing bacteria and leaving skin smooth and clean. It is also not irritating to the skin. It is an inexpensive handy product!

Essential Oils - try lavender, peppermint, lemongrass, frankincense or sandalwood essential oil.

Two cups Apple Cider Vinegar helps to draw out excess uric acid from the body. It can help with joint pain, arthritis, gout and headache relief. It is great for toning your skin also.

Salve

Needed Ingredients:

Beeswax, extra virgin olive oil, castor oil, magnesium oil, peppermint oil, lavender oil and a citrus oil (lemon, orange or grapefruit).

Shred or shave your beeswax if it is bar form ½ oz.
To make a softer salve use less beeswax.
Mix bee wax and carrier oil in a double boiler and melt.
Keep at a low heat.

If you do not have a double boiler you can use a small mason jar over a pan with water in it.

Once melted, remove from heat. You can now add the magnesium, castor and essential oils. Mix quickly and pour into a small jar you would like to store it in.

A smaller jar is best so you can take it on the go with you! Once filled place the jar in the refrigerator to set. Once it is completely hard you can remove it. Shouldn't take more than an hour to firm up.

You can apply this salve to your forehead, temples, neck and shoulders. Anywhere that you have tension and could use relief.

Alternative Options

Daith piercing is an ear piercing that is down in your ears cartilage innermost fold. It is done at a reflex point. It is put into a point that is known to help migraines.

There is no studies done on this but many people have had positive results in getting this piercing. It does not take away all symptoms of migraines but headaches seem to get better for some.

Getting this piercing goes along with acupuncture type treatment. It is believed that this piercing is a totally natural way to relieving chronic headaches.

Essential Oils

Essential oils are a great natural tool to add to your regime for headache relief and prevention.

Peppermint essential oil is wonderful because it creates a cooling sensation when applied to the skin. Great for enhanced blood flow when applied it to the temples or forehead.

Great for migraines and tension headaches. Lavender essential oil is one of the most widely used therapeutic essential oils. It is a wonderful relaxant. It is great for helping with stress and tension.

Helps to relieve anxiety and induce sedation. Lavender essential oil can also help with your sleep cycle. As we talked about before sleep can be a major contributor and help for headaches. Add 5-10 drops of lavender essential oil to a warm bath before bed.

The calming and stimulating effects of both peppermint and lavender essential oils is wonderful in helping relieve headache symptoms. Eucalyptus essential oil is a great cleanser for our body and immune system. It helps to detoxify our bodies of impurities. Can be a great essential oil to use for sinus headaches as it can help open the nasal passages.

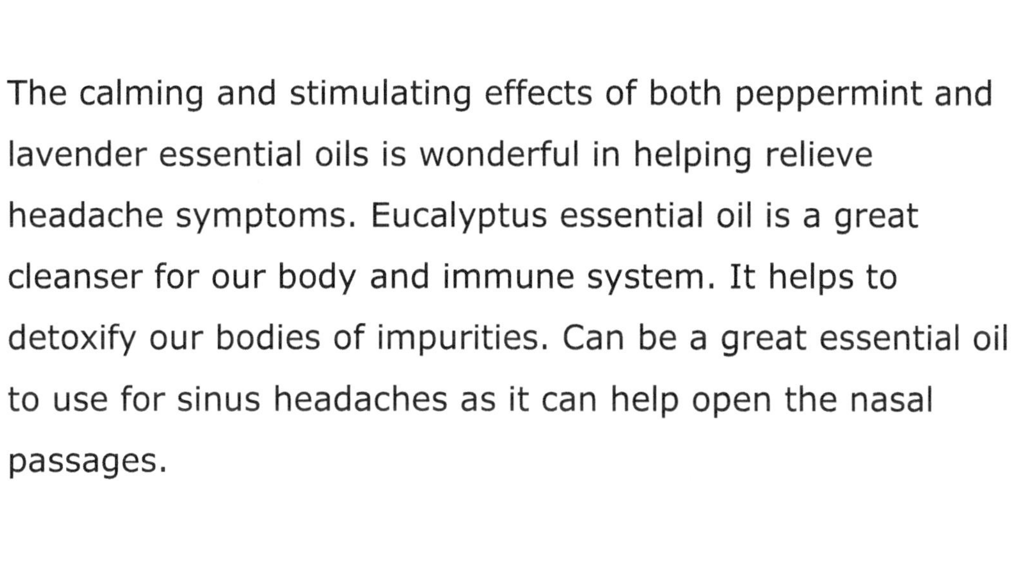

Essential Oils – General Info

Many oils are very potent and can damage your skin. Instead, mix a few drops with a carrier oil like coconut or almond oil before applying it topically to your skin. These carrier oils have a neutral scent and will dilute the more powerful essential oils to the point where they can be applied topically.

Topical Application:

Be sure to avoid applying essential oils to sensitive areas like your ears, around your eyes and mouth and anywhere you have broken or damaged skin. Rub the oil onto your neck, forehead, temples, chest, abdomen, arms, legs, or the bottoms of your feet to feel the oil's benefits.

Aromatic Use:

Essential oil diffusers have become a popular trend in home decor. Ultrasonic diffusers release a hydrating mist into the room that contains the essential oil of your choice.

This is an easy way to use your essential oils because all it requires you to do is breathe Essential oils are the compounds that are extracted from the bark, flowers, leaves, stems, roots, and other parts of plants.

It is also recommended that people carry out an allergy test before using essential oils, as they can cause irritation.

The chemicals in essential oils can interact with the body through being absorbed through the skin into the bloodstream or stimulating areas of the brain through inhalation Applying essential oils to the skin may cause an allergic reaction, skin irritation, and sun sensitivity in some people, so the oils must first be mixed with carrier oil.

It is recommended that children, pregnant women, and breastfeeding women avoid using essential oils, as it is not yet known the effect that they may have on them.

Anyone considering using essential oils should speak to a doctor to discuss the potential benefits and risks.

There is some evidence that essential oils do work and if they do no harm, might improve effectiveness of other treatment approaches or reduce symptoms.

Essential Oil Recipe

Sinus Headache Help

1 drop frankincense

1 drop lavender

1 drop peppermint

Mix in palm of hand with about 1.2 teaspoon of a carrier oil.

Gently massage into forehead, temples and back of neck.

Also, gently rub around sinuses. Take care if keeping it out of

your eyes and nose.

In Conclusion

Having a headache can be miserable. Treating your headache naturally can be very simple. Small changes can lead to big results. Start with one thing for a few days to weeks. Keep track of how it makes you feel. What positive or negative results you get. Keep working through the different options. You can get great results.

The Migraine And Headache Program

Check and discover an natural method that eliminates migraine and frequent headache and gives you an awesome every day.

If you are at the end of your wits migraine and headaches, then discover how fool-proof system can boost the oxygen level in your brain and eliminate your pain with simple, powerful, step by step exercises... permanently curing your migraine and all types of headaches as soon as <u>TODAY!</u>

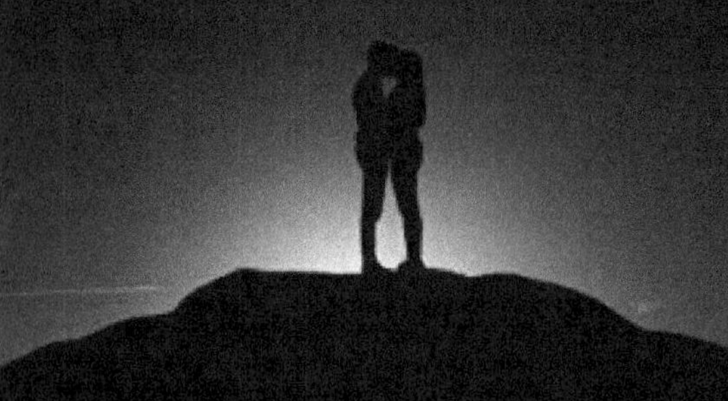

John Zager

HOW
TO CREATE PERFECT
RELATIONSHIP

BECOME THE GUY EVERY WOMAN
DREAMS OF

John Zager

TOTAL CONTROL OF EJACULATION IN 24 HOURS

TAKE 100% CONTROL OF YOUR EJACULATION AND MAKE LOVE FOR AS LONG AS YOU WANT.

John Zager

BE A MAN

IN

BED

HOW TO IMPRESS A GIRL IN BED AND BECOME A GREAT LOVER

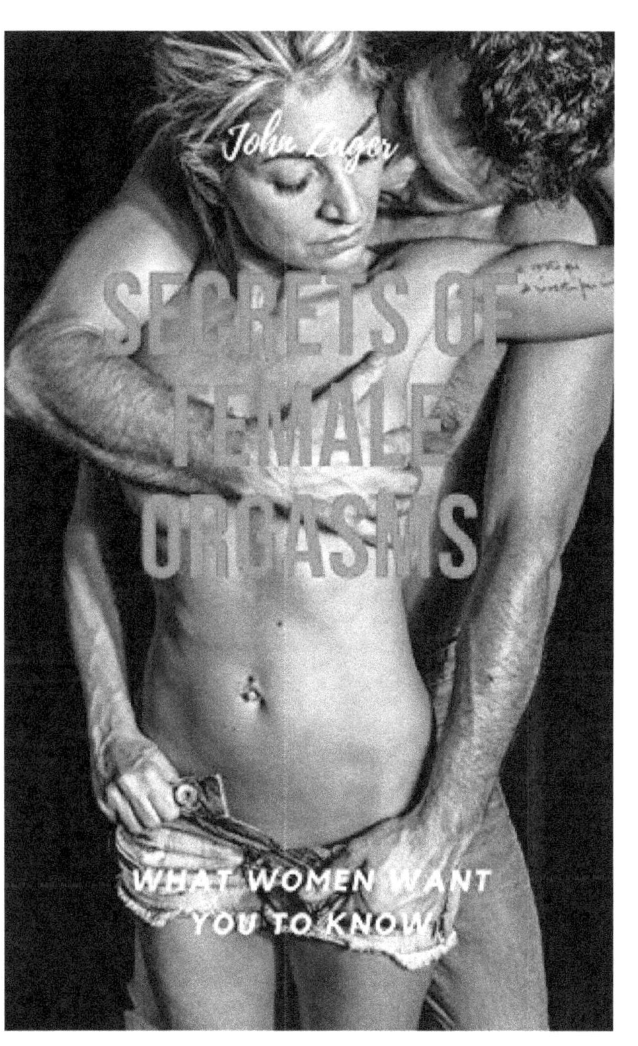

John Zager
SECRETS OF FEMALE ORGASMS
WHAT WOMEN WANT YOU TO KNOW!

MASTER OF REKINDLE

John Zugai

GET 30 AMAZING SKILLS AND MAKE AN IMPRESSION ON EVERY WOMAN

John Zager

THE 10 BEST POSITIONS FOR ORAL SEX

John Zager

MAKE HER SECRET DESIRES COME TRUE

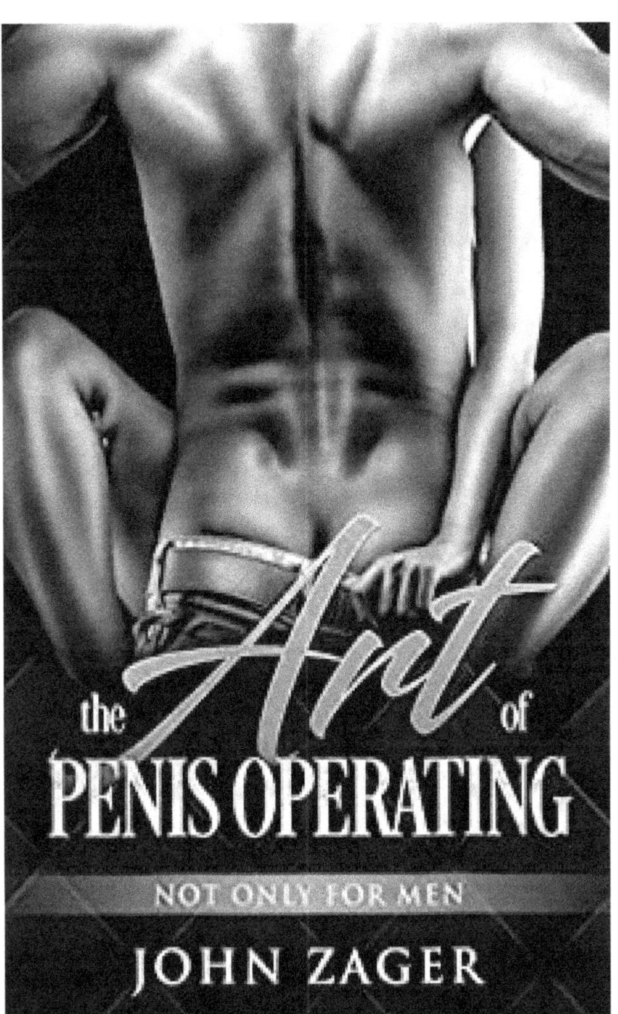

the Art of
PENIS OPERATING
NOT ONLY FOR MEN
JOHN ZAGER

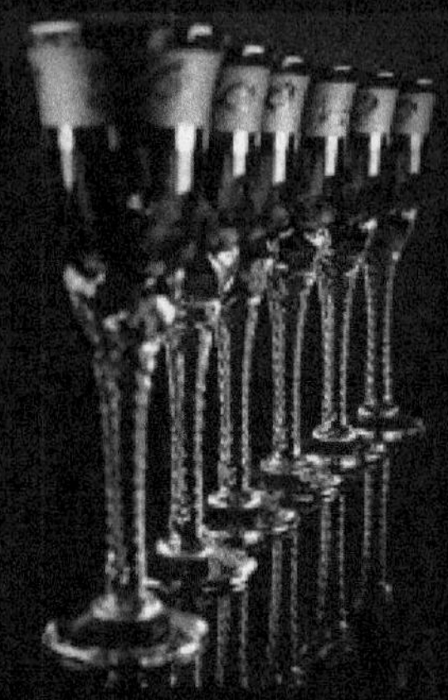

Homemade Liquors

THE UNIQUE RECIPE GUIDE

TOP 12 FRUITS LIQUORS

—

JOHN ZAGER

John Zager

SEVEN FAST STRESS REDUCTION TECHNIQUES

SUPPLEMENTS
EVERYTHING
WHAT YOU NEED
TO KNOW

A GUIDE TO UNDERSTANDING SUPPLEMENTS

JOHN ZAGER

My Notebooks:

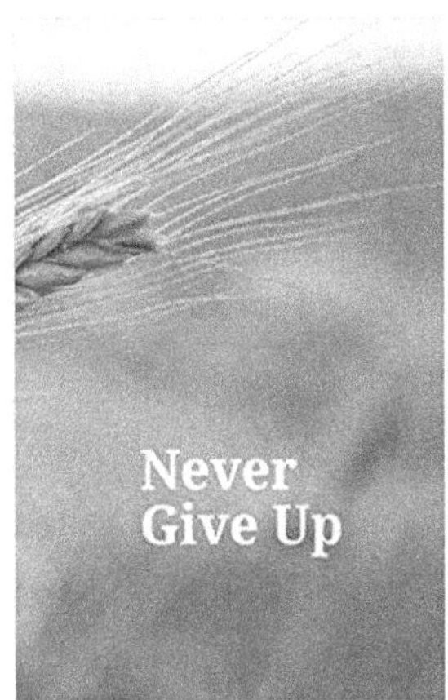

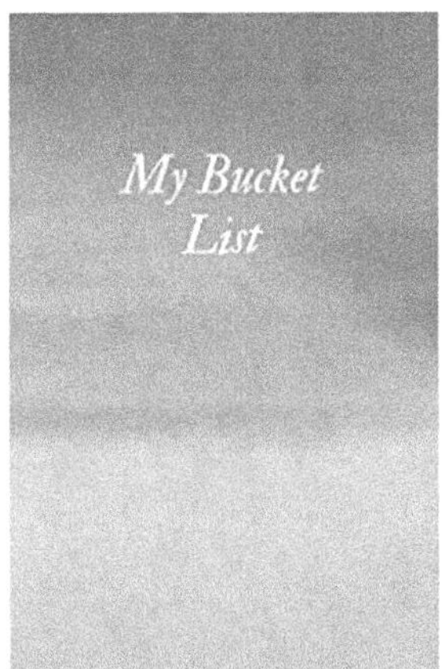

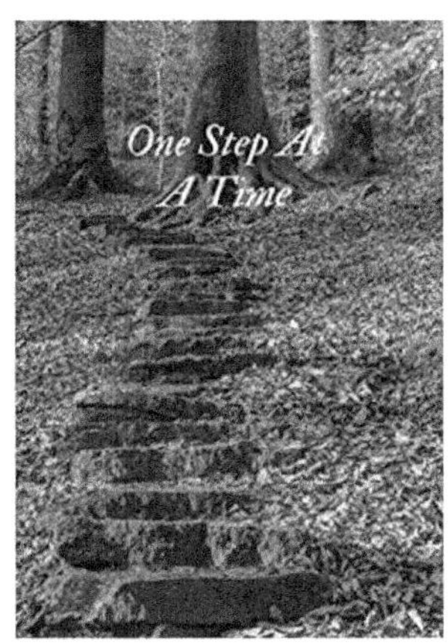

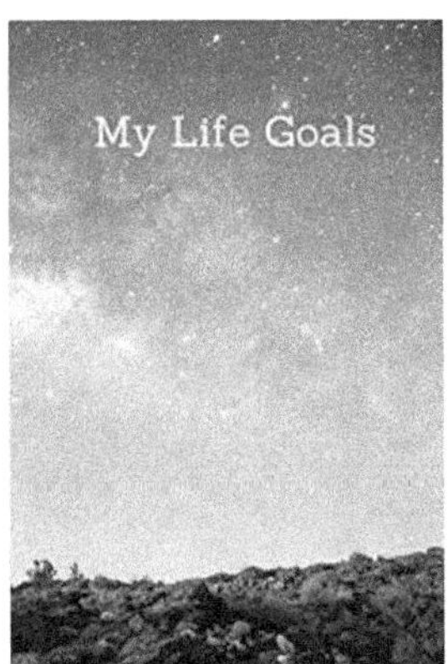

Notes: